Daily Food Journal

This Daily Food Journal Belongs to:

_____

DAY: DATE:

BREAKFAST:	CALORIES
TOTAL BREAKFAST CALORIES:	
LUNCH:	CALORIES
TOTAL LUNCH CALORIES:	
DINNER:	CALORIES
TOTAL DINNER CALORIES:	

The Journey of a thousand miles begins with one step.
- Lao Tzu

SNACKS:	CALORIES

EXERCISE:	DURATION	CALORIES BURNED

GLASSES OF WATER:

CRAVINGS/RESPONSES:

SLEEP:	1 2 3 4 5 6 7 8 9 10
STRESS LEVEL:	1 2 3 4 5 6 7 8 9 10

NOTES:

DAY: DATE:

BREAKFAST:	CALORIES
TOTAL BREAKFAST CALORIES:	
LUNCH:	CALORIES
TOTAL LUNCH CALORIES:	
DINNER:	CALORIES
TOTAL DINNER CALORIES:	

The mountains are calling and I must go.

- John Muir

SNACKS:	CALORIES

EXERCISE:	DURATION	CALORIES BURNED

GLASSES OF WATER:

CRAVINGS/RESPONSES:

SLEEP:	1 2 3 4 5 6 7 8 9 10
STRESS LEVEL:	1 2 3 4 5 6 7 8 9 10

NOTES:

DAY: DATE:

BREAKFAST:	CALORIES
TOTAL BREAKFAST CALORIES:	

LUNCH:	CALORIES
TOTAL LUNCH CALORIES:	

DINNER:	CALORIES
TOTAL DINNER CALORIES:	

Experience is one thing you can't get for nothing.
- Oscar Wilde

SNACKS:	CALORIES

EXERCISE:	DURATION	CALORIES BURNED

GLASSES OF WATER:

CRAVINGS/RESPONSES:

SLEEP:	1 2 3 4 5 6 7 8 9 10
STRESS LEVEL:	1 2 3 4 5 6 7 8 9 10

NOTES:

DAY: DATE:

BREAKFAST:	CALORIES
TOTAL BREAKFAST CALORIES:	

LUNCH:	CALORIES
TOTAL LUNCH CALORIES:	

DINNER:	CALORIES
TOTAL DINNER CALORIES:	

The true mystery of the world is the visible, not the invisible.

— Oscar Wilde

SNACKS:	CALORIES

EXERCISE:	DURATION	CALORIES BURNED

GLASSES OF WATER:

CRAVINGS/RESPONSES:

SLEEP:	1 2 3 4 5 6 7 8 9 10
STRESS LEVEL:	1 2 3 4 5 6 7 8 9 10

NOTES:

DAY: DATE:

BREAKFAST:	CALORIES
TOTAL BREAKFAST CALORIES:	

LUNCH:	CALORIES
TOTAL LUNCH CALORIES:	

DINNER:	CALORIES
TOTAL DINNER CALORIES:	

Cheerfulness is the best promoter of health and is as friendly to the mind as to the body.   - Joseph Addison

SNACKS:	CALORIES

EXERCISE:	DURATION	CALORIES BURNED

GLASSES OF WATER:

CRAVINGS/RESPONSES:

SLEEP:	1 2 3 4 5 6 7 8 9 10
STRESS LEVEL:	1 2 3 4 5 6 7 8 9 10

NOTES:

DAY: DATE:

BREAKFAST:	CALORIES
TOTAL BREAKFAST CALORIES:	
LUNCH:	CALORIES
TOTAL LUNCH CALORIES:	
DINNER:	CALORIES
TOTAL DINNER CALORIES:	

Every noble work is at first impossible.

- Thomas Carlyle

SNACKS:	CALORIES

EXERCISE:	DURATION	CALORIES BURNED

GLASSES OF WATER:

CRAVINGS/RESPONSES:

SLEEP:	1 2 3 4 5 6 7 8 9 10
STRESS LEVEL:	1 2 3 4 5 6 7 8 9 10

NOTES:

DAY: DATE:

BREAKFAST:	CALORIES
TOTAL BREAKFAST CALORIES:	
LUNCH:	CALORIES
TOTAL LUNCH CALORIES:	
DINNER:	CALORIES
TOTAL DINNER CALORIES:	

Everything has beauty, but not everyone sees it.

- Confucius

SNACKS:	CALORIES

EXERCISE:	DURATION	CALORIES BURNED

GLASSES OF WATER:

CRAVINGS/RESPONSES:

SLEEP:	1 2 3 4 5 6 7 8 9 10
STRESS LEVEL:	1 2 3 4 5 6 7 8 9 10

NOTES:

DAY: DATE:

BREAKFAST:	CALORIES
TOTAL BREAKFAST CALORIES:	
LUNCH:	CALORIES
TOTAL LUNCH CALORIES:	
DINNER:	CALORIES
TOTAL DINNER CALORIES:	

It is our attitude at the beginning of a difficult task which, more than anything else, will affect its successful outcome.   - William James

SNACKS:	CALORIES

EXERCISE:	DURATION	CALORIES BURNED

GLASSES OF WATER:

CRAVINGS/RESPONSES:

SLEEP:	1 2 3 4 5 6 7 8 9 10
STRESS LEVEL:	1 2 3 4 5 6 7 8 9 10

NOTES:

DAY: DATE:

BREAKFAST:	CALORIES
TOTAL BREAKFAST CALORIES:	
LUNCH:	CALORIES
TOTAL LUNCH CALORIES:	
DINNER:	CALORIES
TOTAL DINNER CALORIES:	

Perseverance is a great element of success. If you only knock long enough and loud enough at the gate, you are sure to wake up somebody.   - Henry Wadsworth Longfellow

SNACKS:	CALORIES

EXERCISE:	DURATION	CALORIES BURNED

GLASSES OF WATER:

CRAVINGS/RESPONSES:

SLEEP: 1 2 3 4 5 6 7 8 9 10
STRESS LEVEL: 1 2 3 4 5 6 7 8 9 10

NOTES:

DAY: DATE:

BREAKFAST:	CALORIES
TOTAL BREAKFAST CALORIES:	
LUNCH:	CALORIES
TOTAL LUNCH CALORIES:	
DINNER:	CALORIES
TOTAL DINNER CALORIES:	

He who has a why to live can bear almost any how.

- Friedrich Nietzsche

SNACKS:	CALORIES

EXERCISE:	DURATION	CALORIES BURNED

GLASSES OF WATER:

CRAVINGS/RESPONSES:

SLEEP:	1 2 3 4 5 6 7 8 9 10
STRESS LEVEL:	1 2 3 4 5 6 7 8 9 10

NOTES:

DAY: DATE:

BREAKFAST:	CALORIES
TOTAL BREAKFAST CALORIES:	
LUNCH:	CALORIES
TOTAL LUNCH CALORIES:	
DINNER:	CALORIES
TOTAL DINNER CALORIES:	

What we achieve inwardly will change outer reality.

- Plutarch

SNACKS:	CALORIES

EXERCISE:	DURATION	CALORIES BURNED

GLASSES OF WATER:

CRAVINGS/RESPONSES:

SLEEP:	1 2 3 4 5 6 7 8 9 10
STRESS LEVEL:	1 2 3 4 5 6 7 8 9 10

NOTES:

DAY: DATE:

BREAKFAST:	CALORIES
TOTAL BREAKFAST CALORIES:	

LUNCH:	CALORIES
TOTAL LUNCH CALORIES:	

DINNER:	CALORIES
TOTAL DINNER CALORIES:	

Things do not change; we change.

- Henry David Thoreau

SNACKS:	CALORIES

EXERCISE:	DURATION	CALORIES BURNED

GLASSES OF WATER:

CRAVINGS/RESPONSES:

SLEEP:	1 2 3 4 5 6 7 8 9 10
STRESS LEVEL:	1 2 3 4 5 6 7 8 9 10

NOTES:

DAY: DATE:

BREAKFAST:	CALORIES
TOTAL BREAKFAST CALORIES:	
LUNCH:	CALORIES
TOTAL LUNCH CALORIES:	
DINNER:	CALORIES
TOTAL DINNER CALORIES:	

True life is lived when tiny changes occur.

- Leo Tolstoy

SNACKS:	CALORIES

EXERCISE:	DURATION	CALORIES BURNED

GLASSES OF WATER:

CRAVINGS/RESPONSES:

SLEEP:	1 2 3 4 5 6 7 8 9 10
STRESS LEVEL:	1 2 3 4 5 6 7 8 9 10

NOTES:

DAY: DATE:

BREAKFAST:	CALORIES
TOTAL BREAKFAST CALORIES:	

LUNCH:	CALORIES
TOTAL LUNCH CALORIES:	

DINNER:	CALORIES
TOTAL DINNER CALORIES:	

Success consists of getting up just one more time than you fall. - Oliver Goldsmith

SNACKS:	CALORIES

EXERCISE:	DURATION	CALORIES BURNED

GLASSES OF WATER:

CRAVINGS/RESPONSES:

SLEEP:	1 2 3 4 5 6 7 8 9 10
STRESS LEVEL:	1 2 3 4 5 6 7 8 9 10

NOTES:

DAY: DATE:

BREAKFAST:	CALORIES
TOTAL BREAKFAST CALORIES:	
LUNCH:	CALORIES
TOTAL LUNCH CALORIES:	
DINNER:	CALORIES
TOTAL DINNER CALORIES:	

To love oneself is the beginning of a lifelong romance.
- Oscar Wilde

SNACKS:	CALORIES

EXERCISE:	DURATION	CALORIES BURNED

GLASSES OF WATER:

CRAVINGS/RESPONSES:

SLEEP:	1 2 3 4 5 6 7 8 9 10
STRESS LEVEL:	1 2 3 4 5 6 7 8 9 10

NOTES:

DAY: DATE:

BREAKFAST:	CALORIES
TOTAL BREAKFAST CALORIES:	
LUNCH:	CALORIES
TOTAL LUNCH CALORIES:	
DINNER:	CALORIES
TOTAL DINNER CALORIES:	

We are what we repeatedly do. Excellence, then, is not an act, but a habit.   - Aristotle

SNACKS:	CALORIES

EXERCISE:	DURATION	CALORIES BURNED

GLASSES OF WATER:

CRAVINGS/RESPONSES:

SLEEP:	1 2 3 4 5 6 7 8 9 10
STRESS LEVEL:	1 2 3 4 5 6 7 8 9 10

NOTES:

DAY: DATE:

BREAKFAST:	CALORIES
TOTAL BREAKFAST CALORIES:	

LUNCH:	CALORIES
TOTAL LUNCH CALORIES:	

DINNER:	CALORIES
TOTAL DINNER CALORIES:	

Who seeks shall find.

- Sophocles

SNACKS:	CALORIES

EXERCISE:	DURATION	CALORIES BURNED

GLASSES OF WATER:

CRAVINGS/RESPONSES:

SLEEP:	1 2 3 4 5 6 7 8 9 10
STRESS LEVEL:	1 2 3 4 5 6 7 8 9 10

NOTES:

DAY: DATE:

BREAKFAST:	CALORIES
TOTAL BREAKFAST CALORIES:	
LUNCH:	CALORIES
TOTAL LUNCH CALORIES:	
DINNER:	CALORIES
TOTAL DINNER CALORIES:	

Let the beauty of what you love be what you do.

- Rumi

SNACKS:	CALORIES

EXERCISE:	DURATION	CALORIES BURNED

GLASSES OF WATER:

CRAVINGS/RESPONSES:

SLEEP:	1 2 3 4 5 6 7 8 9 10
STRESS LEVEL:	1 2 3 4 5 6 7 8 9 10

NOTES:

DAY: DATE:

BREAKFAST:	CALORIES
TOTAL BREAKFAST CALORIES:	

LUNCH:	CALORIES
TOTAL LUNCH CALORIES:	

DINNER:	CALORIES
TOTAL DINNER CALORIES:	

Just as our eyes need light in order to see, our minds need ideas in order to conceive.   - Nicolas Malebranche

SNACKS:	CALORIES

EXERCISE:	DURATION	CALORIES BURNED

GLASSES OF WATER:

CRAVINGS/RESPONSES:

SLEEP:	1 2 3 4 5 6 7 8 9 10
STRESS LEVEL:	1 2 3 4 5 6 7 8 9 10

NOTES:

DAY: DATE:

BREAKFAST:	CALORIES
TOTAL BREAKFAST CALORIES:	
LUNCH:	CALORIES
TOTAL LUNCH CALORIES:	
DINNER:	CALORIES
TOTAL DINNER CALORIES:	

If you do not change direction, you may end up where you are heading.   - Lao Tzu

SNACKS:	CALORIES

EXERCISE:	DURATION	CALORIES BURNED

GLASSES OF WATER:

CRAVINGS/RESPONSES:

SLEEP:	1 2 3 4 5 6 7 8 9 10
STRESS LEVEL:	1 2 3 4 5 6 7 8 9 10

NOTES:

DAY: DATE:

BREAKFAST:	CALORIES
TOTAL BREAKFAST CALORIES:	

LUNCH:	CALORIES
TOTAL LUNCH CALORIES:	

DINNER:	CALORIES
TOTAL DINNER CALORIES:	

They succeed, because they think they can.

- Virgil

SNACKS:	CALORIES

EXERCISE:	DURATION	CALORIES BURNED

GLASSES OF WATER:

CRAVINGS/RESPONSES:

SLEEP:	1 2 3 4 5 6 7 8 9 10
STRESS LEVEL:	1 2 3 4 5 6 7 8 9 10

NOTES:

DAY: DATE:

BREAKFAST:	CALORIES
TOTAL BREAKFAST CALORIES:	
LUNCH:	CALORIES
TOTAL LUNCH CALORIES:	
DINNER:	CALORIES
TOTAL DINNER CALORIES:	

If we learn not humility, we learn nothing.

- John Jewel

SNACKS:	CALORIES

EXERCISE:	DURATION	CALORIES BURNED

GLASSES OF WATER:

CRAVINGS/RESPONSES:

SLEEP:	1 2 3 4 5 6 7 8 9 10
STRESS LEVEL:	1 2 3 4 5 6 7 8 9 10

NOTES:

DAY: DATE:

BREAKFAST:	CALORIES
TOTAL BREAKFAST CALORIES:	

LUNCH:	CALORIES
TOTAL LUNCH CALORIES:	

DINNER:	CALORIES
TOTAL DINNER CALORIES:	

This world is but a canvas to our imagination.
- Henry David Thoreau

SNACKS:	CALORIES

EXERCISE:	DURATION	CALORIES BURNED

GLASSES OF WATER:

CRAVINGS/RESPONSES:

SLEEP:	1 2 3 4 5 6 7 8 9 10
STRESS LEVEL:	1 2 3 4 5 6 7 8 9 10

NOTES:

DAY: DATE:

BREAKFAST:	CALORIES
TOTAL BREAKFAST CALORIES:	

LUNCH:	CALORIES
TOTAL LUNCH CALORIES:	

DINNER:	CALORIES
TOTAL DINNER CALORIES:	

That man is a success who has lived well, laughed often and loved much.   - Robert Louis Stevenson

SNACKS:	CALORIES

EXERCISE:	DURATION	CALORIES BURNED

GLASSES OF WATER:

CRAVINGS/RESPONSES:

SLEEP:	1 2 3 4 5 6 7 8 9 10
STRESS LEVEL:	1 2 3 4 5 6 7 8 9 10

NOTES:

DAY: DATE:

BREAKFAST:	CALORIES
TOTAL BREAKFAST CALORIES:	

LUNCH:	CALORIES
TOTAL LUNCH CALORIES:	

DINNER:	CALORIES
TOTAL DINNER CALORIES:	

Don't judge each day by the harvest you reap but by the seeds that you plant.   - Robert Louis Stevenson

SNACKS:	CALORIES

EXERCISE:	DURATION	CALORIES BURNED

GLASSES OF WATER:

CRAVINGS/RESPONSES:

SLEEP:	1 2 3 4 5 6 7 8 9 10
STRESS LEVEL:	1 2 3 4 5 6 7 8 9 10

NOTES:

DAY: DATE:

BREAKFAST:	CALORIES
TOTAL BREAKFAST CALORIES:	
LUNCH:	CALORIES
TOTAL LUNCH CALORIES:	
DINNER:	CALORIES
TOTAL DINNER CALORIES:	

A lie can travel half way around the world while the truth is putting on its shoes.   - Charles Spurgeon

SNACKS:	CALORIES

EXERCISE:	DURATION	CALORIES BURNED

GLASSES OF WATER:

CRAVINGS/RESPONSES:

SLEEP:	1 2 3 4 5 6 7 8 9 10
STRESS LEVEL:	1 2 3 4 5 6 7 8 9 10

NOTES:

DAY: DATE:

BREAKFAST:	CALORIES
TOTAL BREAKFAST CALORIES:	
LUNCH:	CALORIES
TOTAL LUNCH CALORIES:	
DINNER:	CALORIES
TOTAL DINNER CALORIES:	

What we achieve inwardly will change outer reality.
- Plutarch

SNACKS:	CALORIES

EXERCISE:	DURATION	CALORIES BURNED

GLASSES OF WATER:

CRAVINGS/RESPONSES:

SLEEP:	1 2 3 4 5 6 7 8 9 10
STRESS LEVEL:	1 2 3 4 5 6 7 8 9 10

NOTES:

DAY: DATE:

BREAKFAST:	CALORIES
TOTAL BREAKFAST CALORIES:	
LUNCH:	CALORIES
TOTAL LUNCH CALORIES:	
DINNER:	CALORIES
TOTAL DINNER CALORIES:	

To every action there is always opposed an equal reaction.
- Isaac Newton

SNACKS:	CALORIES

EXERCISE:	DURATION	CALORIES BURNED

GLASSES OF WATER:

CRAVINGS/RESPONSES:

SLEEP:	1 2 3 4 5 6 7 8 9 10
STRESS LEVEL:	1 2 3 4 5 6 7 8 9 10

NOTES:

DAY: DATE:

BREAKFAST:	CALORIES
TOTAL BREAKFAST CALORIES:	
LUNCH:	CALORIES
TOTAL LUNCH CALORIES:	
DINNER:	CALORIES
TOTAL DINNER CALORIES:	

Man's greatness lies in his power of thought.

- Blaise Pascal

SNACKS:	CALORIES

EXERCISE:	DURATION	CALORIES BURNED

GLASSES OF WATER:

CRAVINGS/RESPONSES:

SLEEP:	1 2 3 4 5 6 7 8 9 10
STRESS LEVEL:	1 2 3 4 5 6 7 8 9 10

NOTES:

DAY: DATE:

BREAKFAST:	CALORIES
TOTAL BREAKFAST CALORIES:	
LUNCH:	CALORIES
TOTAL LUNCH CALORIES:	
DINNER:	CALORIES
TOTAL DINNER CALORIES:	

Nothing would be done at all if one waited until one could do it so well that no one could find fault with it.

- John Henry Newman

SNACKS:	CALORIES

EXERCISE:	DURATION	CALORIES BURNED

GLASSES OF WATER:

CRAVINGS/RESPONSES:

SLEEP:	1 2 3 4 5 6 7 8 9 10
STRESS LEVEL:	1 2 3 4 5 6 7 8 9 10

NOTES:

DAY: DATE:

BREAKFAST:	CALORIES
TOTAL BREAKFAST CALORIES:	
LUNCH:	CALORIES
TOTAL LUNCH CALORIES:	
DINNER:	CALORIES
TOTAL DINNER CALORIES:	

That which we obtain too easily, we esteem too lightly.

- Thomas Paine

SNACKS:	CALORIES

EXERCISE:	DURATION	CALORIES BURNED

GLASSES OF WATER:

CRAVINGS/RESPONSES:

SLEEP:	1 2 3 4 5 6 7 8 9 10
STRESS LEVEL:	1 2 3 4 5 6 7 8 9 10

NOTES:

DAY: DATE:

BREAKFAST:	CALORIES
TOTAL BREAKFAST CALORIES:	
LUNCH:	CALORIES
TOTAL LUNCH CALORIES:	
DINNER:	CALORIES
TOTAL DINNER CALORIES:	

Creativity is not the finding of a thing, but the making something out of it after it is found.

— James Russell Lowell

SNACKS:	CALORIES

EXERCISE:	DURATION	CALORIES BURNED

GLASSES OF WATER:

CRAVINGS/RESPONSES:

SLEEP:	1 2 3 4 5 6 7 8 9 10
STRESS LEVEL:	1 2 3 4 5 6 7 8 9 10

NOTES:

DAY: DATE:

BREAKFAST:	CALORIES
TOTAL BREAKFAST CALORIES:	

LUNCH:	CALORIES
TOTAL LUNCH CALORIES:	

DINNER:	CALORIES
TOTAL DINNER CALORIES:	

Imagination is the eye of the soul.

- Joseph Joubert

SNACKS:	CALORIES

EXERCISE:	DURATION	CALORIES BURNED

GLASSES OF WATER:

CRAVINGS/RESPONSES:

SLEEP:	1 2 3 4 5 6 7 8 9 10
STRESS LEVEL:	1 2 3 4 5 6 7 8 9 10

NOTES:

DAY: DATE:

BREAKFAST:	CALORIES
TOTAL BREAKFAST CALORIES:	

LUNCH:	CALORIES
TOTAL LUNCH CALORIES:	

DINNER:	CALORIES
TOTAL DINNER CALORIES:	

The final proof of greatness lies in being able to endure criticism without resentment.

- Elbert Hubbard

SNACKS:	CALORIES

EXERCISE:	DURATION	CALORIES BURNED

GLASSES OF WATER:

CRAVINGS/RESPONSES:

SLEEP:	1 2 3 4 5 6 7 8 9 10
STRESS LEVEL:	1 2 3 4 5 6 7 8 9 10

NOTES:

DAY: DATE:

BREAKFAST:	CALORIES
TOTAL BREAKFAST CALORIES:	

LUNCH:	CALORIES
TOTAL LUNCH CALORIES:	

DINNER:	CALORIES
TOTAL DINNER CALORIES:	

All things are difficult before they are easy.

- Thomas Fuller

SNACKS:	CALORIES

EXERCISE:	DURATION	CALORIES BURNED

GLASSES OF WATER:

CRAVINGS/RESPONSES:

SLEEP:	1 2 3 4 5 6 7 8 9 10
STRESS LEVEL:	1 2 3 4 5 6 7 8 9 10

NOTES:

DAY: DATE:

BREAKFAST:	CALORIES
TOTAL BREAKFAST CALORIES:	
LUNCH:	CALORIES
TOTAL LUNCH CALORIES:	
DINNER:	CALORIES
TOTAL DINNER CALORIES:	

The key is to keep company only with people who uplift you, whose presence calls forth your best.

- Epictetus

SNACKS:	CALORIES

EXERCISE:	DURATION	CALORIES BURNED

GLASSES OF WATER:

CRAVINGS/RESPONSES:

SLEEP:	1 2 3 4 5 6 7 8 9 10
STRESS LEVEL:	1 2 3 4 5 6 7 8 9 10

NOTES:

DAY: DATE:

BREAKFAST:	CALORIES
TOTAL BREAKFAST CALORIES:	
LUNCH:	CALORIES
TOTAL LUNCH CALORIES:	
DINNER:	CALORIES
TOTAL DINNER CALORIES:	

Trials teach us what we are; they dig up the soil, and let us see what we are made of. - Charles Spurgeon

SNACKS:	CALORIES

EXERCISE:	DURATION	CALORIES BURNED

GLASSES OF WATER:

CRAVINGS/RESPONSES:

SLEEP:	1 2 3 4 5 6 7 8 9 10
STRESS LEVEL:	1 2 3 4 5 6 7 8 9 10

NOTES:

DAY: DATE:

BREAKFAST:	CALORIES
TOTAL BREAKFAST CALORIES:	
LUNCH:	CALORIES
TOTAL LUNCH CALORIES:	
DINNER:	CALORIES
TOTAL DINNER CALORIES:	

We cannot teach people anything; we can only help them discover it within themselves.   - Galileo Galilei

SNACKS:	CALORIES

EXERCISE:	DURATION	CALORIES BURNED

GLASSES OF WATER:

CRAVINGS/RESPONSES:

SLEEP:	1 2 3 4 5 6 7 8 9 10
STRESS LEVEL:	1 2 3 4 5 6 7 8 9 10

NOTES:

DAY: DATE:

BREAKFAST:	CALORIES
TOTAL BREAKFAST CALORIES:	

LUNCH:	CALORIES
TOTAL LUNCH CALORIES:	

DINNER:	CALORIES
TOTAL DINNER CALORIES:	

Our life is what our thoughts make it.

- Marcus Aurelius

SNACKS:	CALORIES

EXERCISE:	DURATION	CALORIES BURNED

GLASSES OF WATER:

CRAVINGS/RESPONSES:

SLEEP:	1 2 3 4 5 6 7 8 9 10
STRESS LEVEL:	1 2 3 4 5 6 7 8 9 10

NOTES:

DAY: DATE:

BREAKFAST:	CALORIES
TOTAL BREAKFAST CALORIES:	
LUNCH:	CALORIES
TOTAL LUNCH CALORIES:	
DINNER:	CALORIES
TOTAL DINNER CALORIES:	

There is nothing on this earth more to be prized than true friendship.   - Thomas Aquinas

SNACKS:	CALORIES

EXERCISE:	DURATION	CALORIES BURNED

GLASSES OF WATER:

CRAVINGS/RESPONSES:

SLEEP:	1 2 3 4 5 6 7 8 9 10
STRESS LEVEL:	1 2 3 4 5 6 7 8 9 10

NOTES:

DAY: DATE:

BREAKFAST:	CALORIES
TOTAL BREAKFAST CALORIES:	
LUNCH:	CALORIES
TOTAL LUNCH CALORIES:	
DINNER:	CALORIES
TOTAL DINNER CALORIES:	

The level of our success is limited only by our imagination and no act of kindness, however small, is ever wasted.

- Aesop

SNACKS:	CALORIES

EXERCISE:	DURATION	CALORIES BURNED

GLASSES OF WATER:

CRAVINGS/RESPONSES:

SLEEP:	1 2 3 4 5 6 7 8 9 10
STRESS LEVEL:	1 2 3 4 5 6 7 8 9 10

NOTES:

DAY: DATE:

BREAKFAST:	CALORIES
TOTAL BREAKFAST CALORIES:	
LUNCH:	CALORIES
TOTAL LUNCH CALORIES:	
DINNER:	CALORIES
TOTAL DINNER CALORIES:	

Our greatest glory is not in never falling, but in rising every time we fall.   - Confucius

SNACKS:	CALORIES

EXERCISE:	DURATION	CALORIES BURNED

GLASSES OF WATER:

CRAVINGS/RESPONSES:

SLEEP:	1 2 3 4 5 6 7 8 9 10
STRESS LEVEL:	1 2 3 4 5 6 7 8 9 10

NOTES:

DAY: DATE:

BREAKFAST:	CALORIES
TOTAL BREAKFAST CALORIES:	

LUNCH:	CALORIES
TOTAL LUNCH CALORIES:	

DINNER:	CALORIES
TOTAL DINNER CALORIES:	

Life consists not in holding good cards but in playing those you hold well.   - Josh Billings

SNACKS:	CALORIES

EXERCISE:	DURATION	CALORIES BURNED

GLASSES OF WATER:

CRAVINGS/RESPONSES:

SLEEP:	1　2　3　4　5　6　7　8　9　10
STRESS LEVEL:	1　2　3　4　5　6　7　8　9　10

NOTES:

DAY: DATE:

BREAKFAST:	CALORIES
TOTAL BREAKFAST CALORIES:	

LUNCH:	CALORIES
TOTAL LUNCH CALORIES:	

DINNER:	CALORIES
TOTAL DINNER CALORIES:	

Wisdom begins in wonder.

- Socrates

SNACKS:	CALORIES

EXERCISE:	DURATION	CALORIES BURNED

GLASSES OF WATER: 🥛 🥛 🥛 🥛 🥛 🥛 🥛 🥛 🥛 🥛

CRAVINGS/RESPONSES:

SLEEP:	1 2 3 4 5 6 7 8 9 10
STRESS LEVEL:	1 2 3 4 5 6 7 8 9 10

NOTES:

DAY: DATE:

BREAKFAST:	CALORIES
TOTAL BREAKFAST CALORIES:	
LUNCH:	CALORIES
TOTAL LUNCH CALORIES:	
DINNER:	CALORIES
TOTAL DINNER CALORIES:	

Life in abundance comes only through great love.
- Elbert Hubbard

SNACKS:	CALORIES

EXERCISE:	DURATION	CALORIES BURNED

GLASSES OF WATER:

CRAVINGS/RESPONSES:

SLEEP:	1 2 3 4 5 6 7 8 9 10
STRESS LEVEL:	1 2 3 4 5 6 7 8 9 10

NOTES:

DAY: DATE:

BREAKFAST:	CALORIES
TOTAL BREAKFAST CALORIES:	
LUNCH:	CALORIES
TOTAL LUNCH CALORIES:	
DINNER:	CALORIES
TOTAL DINNER CALORIES:	

I dwell in possibility.

- Emily Dickinson

SNACKS:	CALORIES

EXERCISE:	DURATION	CALORIES BURNED

GLASSES OF WATER:

CRAVINGS/RESPONSES:

SLEEP:	1 2 3 4 5 6 7 8 9 10
STRESS LEVEL:	1 2 3 4 5 6 7 8 9 10

NOTES:

DAY: DATE:

BREAKFAST:	CALORIES
TOTAL BREAKFAST CALORIES:	

LUNCH:	CALORIES
TOTAL LUNCH CALORIES:	

DINNER:	CALORIES
TOTAL DINNER CALORIES:	

Appreciation is a wonderful thing: It makes what is excellent in others belong to us as well.   - Voltaire

SNACKS:	CALORIES

EXERCISE:	DURATION	CALORIES BURNED

GLASSES OF WATER:

CRAVINGS/RESPONSES:

SLEEP:	1 2 3 4 5 6 7 8 9 10
STRESS LEVEL:	1 2 3 4 5 6 7 8 9 10

NOTES:

DAY: DATE:

BREAKFAST:	CALORIES
TOTAL BREAKFAST CALORIES:	

LUNCH:	CALORIES
TOTAL LUNCH CALORIES:	

DINNER:	CALORIES
TOTAL DINNER CALORIES:	

When unhappy, one doubts everything; when happy, one doubts nothing.   - Joseph Roux

SNACKS:	CALORIES

EXERCISE:	DURATION	CALORIES BURNED

GLASSES OF WATER:

CRAVINGS/RESPONSES:

SLEEP:	1 2 3 4 5 6 7 8 9 10
STRESS LEVEL:	1 2 3 4 5 6 7 8 9 10

NOTES:

DAY:　　　　　　　　　　DATE:

BREAKFAST:	CALORIES
TOTAL BREAKFAST CALORIES:	

LUNCH:	CALORIES
TOTAL LUNCH CALORIES:	

DINNER:	CALORIES
TOTAL DINNER CALORIES:	

Good actions give strength to ourselves and inspire good actions in others.　　　　　　　　　　- Plato

SNACKS:	CALORIES

EXERCISE:	DURATION	CALORIES BURNED

GLASSES OF WATER:

CRAVINGS/RESPONSES:

SLEEP:	1 2 3 4 5 6 7 8 9 10
STRESS LEVEL:	1 2 3 4 5 6 7 8 9 10

NOTES:

DAY: DATE:

BREAKFAST:	CALORIES
TOTAL BREAKFAST CALORIES:	

LUNCH:	CALORIES
TOTAL LUNCH CALORIES:	

DINNER:	CALORIES
TOTAL DINNER CALORIES:	

Our best successes often come after our greatest disappointments.   - Henry Ward Beecher

SNACKS:	CALORIES

EXERCISE:	DURATION	CALORIES BURNED

GLASSES OF WATER:

CRAVINGS/RESPONSES:

SLEEP:	1 2 3 4 5 6 7 8 9 10
STRESS LEVEL:	1 2 3 4 5 6 7 8 9 10

NOTES:

DAY: DATE:

BREAKFAST:	CALORIES
TOTAL BREAKFAST CALORIES:	
LUNCH:	CALORIES
TOTAL LUNCH CALORIES:	
DINNER:	CALORIES
TOTAL DINNER CALORIES:	

The future is purchased by the present.

- Samuel Johnson

SNACKS:	CALORIES

EXERCISE:	DURATION	CALORIES BURNED

GLASSES OF WATER:

CRAVINGS/RESPONSES:

SLEEP:	1 2 3 4 5 6 7 8 9 10
STRESS LEVEL:	1 2 3 4 5 6 7 8 9 10

NOTES:

DAY: DATE:

BREAKFAST:	CALORIES
TOTAL BREAKFAST CALORIES:	
LUNCH:	CALORIES
TOTAL LUNCH CALORIES:	
DINNER:	CALORIES
TOTAL DINNER CALORIES:	

Remember when life's path is steep to keep your mind even.
— Horace

SNACKS:	CALORIES

EXERCISE:	DURATION	CALORIES BURNED

GLASSES OF WATER:

CRAVINGS/RESPONSES:

SLEEP:	1 2 3 4 5 6 7 8 9 10
STRESS LEVEL:	1 2 3 4 5 6 7 8 9 10

NOTES:

DAY: DATE:

BREAKFAST:	CALORIES
TOTAL BREAKFAST CALORIES:	

LUNCH:	CALORIES
TOTAL LUNCH CALORIES:	

DINNER:	CALORIES
TOTAL DINNER CALORIES:	

The best preparation for tomorrow is to do today's work superbly well.   - William Osler

SNACKS:	CALORIES

EXERCISE:	DURATION	CALORIES BURNED

GLASSES OF WATER:

CRAVINGS/RESPONSES:

SLEEP:	1 2 3 4 5 6 7 8 9 10
STRESS LEVEL:	1 2 3 4 5 6 7 8 9 10

NOTES:

DAY: DATE:

BREAKFAST:	CALORIES
TOTAL BREAKFAST CALORIES:	
LUNCH:	CALORIES
TOTAL LUNCH CALORIES:	
DINNER:	CALORIES
TOTAL DINNER CALORIES:	

Genius is the ability to renew one's emotions in daily experience.
— Paul Cezanne

SNACKS:	CALORIES

EXERCISE:	DURATION	CALORIES BURNED

GLASSES OF WATER:

CRAVINGS/RESPONSES:

SLEEP:	1 2 3 4 5 6 7 8 9 10
STRESS LEVEL:	1 2 3 4 5 6 7 8 9 10

NOTES:

DAY: DATE:

BREAKFAST:	CALORIES
TOTAL BREAKFAST CALORIES:	

LUNCH:	CALORIES
TOTAL LUNCH CALORIES:	

DINNER:	CALORIES
TOTAL DINNER CALORIES:	

A gentle word, a kind look, a good-natured smile can work wonders and accomplish miracles.   - William Hazlitt

SNACKS:	CALORIES

EXERCISE:	DURATION	CALORIES BURNED

GLASSES OF WATER:

CRAVINGS/RESPONSES:

SLEEP:	1 2 3 4 5 6 7 8 9 10
STRESS LEVEL:	1 2 3 4 5 6 7 8 9 10

NOTES:

DAY: DATE:

BREAKFAST:	CALORIES
TOTAL BREAKFAST CALORIES:	

LUNCH:	CALORIES
TOTAL LUNCH CALORIES:	

DINNER:	CALORIES
TOTAL DINNER CALORIES:	

If you want the present to be different from the past, study the past.   - Baruch Spinoza

SNACKS:	CALORIES

EXERCISE:	DURATION	CALORIES BURNED

GLASSES OF WATER: 🥛🥛🥛🥛🥛🥛🥛🥛🥛

CRAVINGS/RESPONSES:

SLEEP:	1 2 3 4 5 6 7 8 9 10
STRESS LEVEL:	1 2 3 4 5 6 7 8 9 10

NOTES:

DAY: DATE:

BREAKFAST:	CALORIES
TOTAL BREAKFAST CALORIES:	
LUNCH:	CALORIES
TOTAL LUNCH CALORIES:	
DINNER:	CALORIES
TOTAL DINNER CALORIES:	

Begin, be bold and venture to be wise.

- Horace

SNACKS:	CALORIES

EXERCISE:	DURATION	CALORIES BURNED

GLASSES OF WATER:

CRAVINGS/RESPONSES:

SLEEP:	1 2 3 4 5 6 7 8 9 10
STRESS LEVEL:	1 2 3 4 5 6 7 8 9 10

NOTES:

DAY: DATE:

BREAKFAST:	CALORIES
TOTAL BREAKFAST CALORIES:	
LUNCH:	CALORIES
TOTAL LUNCH CALORIES:	
DINNER:	CALORIES
TOTAL DINNER CALORIES:	

He who knows that enough is enough will always have enough.   - Lao Tzu

SNACKS:	CALORIES

EXERCISE:	DURATION	CALORIES BURNED

GLASSES OF WATER:

CRAVINGS/RESPONSES:

SLEEP:	1 2 3 4 5 6 7 8 9 10
STRESS LEVEL:	1 2 3 4 5 6 7 8 9 10

NOTES:

DAY: DATE:

BREAKFAST:	CALORIES
TOTAL BREAKFAST CALORIES:	
LUNCH:	CALORIES
TOTAL LUNCH CALORIES:	
DINNER:	CALORIES
TOTAL DINNER CALORIES:	

Never give up, for that is just the place and time that the tide will turn. - Harriet Beecher Stowe

SNACKS:	CALORIES

EXERCISE:	DURATION	CALORIES BURNED

GLASSES OF WATER:

CRAVINGS/RESPONSES:

SLEEP:	1 2 3 4 5 6 7 8 9 10
STRESS LEVEL:	1 2 3 4 5 6 7 8 9 10

NOTES:

Shredded Wheat - 10 — 70 cals
Cornflakes   green tub   113 cals.

250 gms milk   235

Yogurt & Prunes   150

Wheat Crackers   22 each.
Apple   52